Ketogenic Diet

For
Ultimate Weight Loss

More Delicious Recipes to
Lose Belly Fat Fast!

Steven Ballinger

Table of Contents

Important Insight

For people who are interested in losing weight the right way – slowly but steadily, so that it stays off over time – then cutting carbs has proven to be a highly effective way to do it.

The ketogenic diet is one plan that has worked for many people who couldn't lose weight any other way. The ketogenic diet started out as a dietary plan for people suffering from epilepsy. It goes against what used to be traditional weight loss advice, as the diet contains fats and proteins. The principle behind the diet is that it makes your body run on fat as opposed to carbohydrate as a primary fuel.

In most cases, the body turns the carbohydrates from food into glucose, which it then sends around the body to fuel cellular function. However, when your diet contains only a scant amounts of carbohydrates, your liver starts turning fat into ketone bodies and fatty acids.

The ketone bodies move into the brain and serve as an energy source, replacing glucose. It is the higher level of ketone bodies in the bloodstream, leading to a condition called ketosis that refers to your body's new system of fuel.

This book contains a number of recipes that you can use as you change to the ketogenic diet. It can be difficult to change to a new system of nutrition; not only do our bodies resist change initially, but given our hectic lifestyles, cooking dinner is often the last thing we want to do
.

Armed with these recipes, you can manage your diet, instead of letting your diet manage you. The end result will not just be weight loss: you will feel higher levels of energy, and you will feel better overall. The fact that your clothes fit better will just be (low-calorie) icing on the (very low carb) cake.

Enjoy this assortment of recipes designed to take you throughout your nutritional day.

1: Breakfast: The Most Important Meal of the Day

You might be tempted to jump right over breakfast during your dietary day, thinking that cutting those calories out of your eating will help you lose weight. Unfortunately, this is an idea that can actually backfire.

There are a couple of reasons for this: first, your metabolism will slow down to a crawl, and then you'll eat more than you normally would at your next meal.

If you give in and eat some snacks, you're likely to grab something high in carbs. There are some studies that indicate that we add body fat in higher amounts when we eat fewer meals of larger size.

The research is a little mixed here, but it is emphatic about the metabolic boost that breakfast gives you, especially when it's a meal higher in protein and fats.

High in protein and fats, you say? That sounds like a ketogenic plan! Check out some of these recipes.

Principle #1: Learn to love the quiche

When you eat breakfast, you want it to be a filling meal so that you are not tempted to snack throughout the day. Study after study shows that if you eat a satisfying breakfast, you will regulate your consumption of food the rest of the day much more effectively.

So why quiche? It's easy to make, easy to freeze and store for the week, and it combines eggs, cheese and other proteins that will stay in your stomach longer. Too many breakfast foods are high in carbs; by choosing quiche, you have everything on the ketogenic plan.

Most of these recipes are crustless, which means that your carb count will be low. Just remember to butter the pan so that the mixture doesn't stick when it's done. Make one of these on Sunday and just cut out a slice each day throughout the week for breakfast.

Stick with medium cheese that melts easily, like Havarti, Muenster, Swiss and cheddar. Harder cheeses like Romano and Parmesan don't melt as well, and they also have a lot of salt.

Cheese and Onion Quiche

This recipe yields two quiches, each in a 10-inch quiche pan or a deep pie pan.

Ingredients:
5-6 cups shredded Muenster and/or Colby jack cheese, divided in half
2 tablespoons butter plus more for greasing pans
1 large white onion, finely chopped
12 large eggs, preferably organic or free range eggs
2 cups heavy cream
1 tsp salt
1 tsp ground black pepper
2 tsp dried thyme

Directions:

1. Preheat your oven to 350 F.

2. Melt the butter in a skillet that is over medium-low heat. When it has melted, add in the veggies and sauté until you see soft, translucent onions. Take out of the pan and allow cooling.

3. Butter the pans, and cover the bottom of each pan, and add half of the veggie mixture to

both pans, making an even layer on top of the cheese.

4. Crack a dozen eggs into a large mixing bowl. Add the spices and cream before whisking until they are frothy and well mixed. Half of the mixture goes into each pan. Spread the vegetables and cheese evenly with the cream and egg mixture.

5. Put the pans into your oven, leaving a gap of about an inch between them. Bake until they are puffy and set, with a touch of gold in the center. Stick a knife into the center of one and pull it out; if it is clean, the quiche is finished.

6. Cut the quiche into six equally sized pieces. You can serve now or place in the refrigerator (for up to a week) or the freezer (for up to two weeks).

Nutrition:
Each serving (6 servings) has 16 grams of protein, 382 calories, 5 grams of carbs, 1 grab of fiber, and 33 grams of fat.

Want to mix it up?

There are many ways to add variety to your quiche repertoire. If you want a little meat, consider adding sausage or bacon to the quiche as well. To add bacon, just put a dozen slices of raw bacon onto a cookie sheet, and bake them at 350 F for 20 minutes or until the pieces are just a bit crispy. Then, allow them to cool before putting the pieces into a food processor.
This only adds 8 calories to each serving, but it adds 3 grams of protein and no carbs.

To add sausage, put six ounces of pork breakfast sausage into a skillet and cook it until it is done. Allow to cool and then crumble before stirring it into the cream and egg mixture that appears in Step 4 up there. This keeps your nutritional information almost identical.

What if you want to add some vegetables? Just about any choice that is low in carbs will work. Just throw your broccoli, bell peppers, carrots, celery, summer squash or other veggie into the food processor. Then, add this to your sauté pan in Step 2 above. For each cup of vegetables that you add, you'll get one more gram of carbohydrates in each serving.

The good thing about quiche is that you can add just about anything you want. Smoked ham? Check. Shrimp? Check. Smoked sausage? Check. Take a look at the nutrition labels on anything you want to add, and make sure that you're not putting in any sneaky carbs (you'll want to stay away from honey cured hams, for example).

The focus on a ketogenic diet is to boost proteins and fats while reducing the number of carbs you're taking in, because you're want to teach your body to burn fats instead of carbohydrates.

If you get in the habit of cooking and freezing one of these quiches on Sunday, then you'll have breakfast all week long. You'll also have the tasty goodness of a warm, filling breakfast without having to use any other cooking utensils during the week besides your microwave oven. It's a win-win situation every day of the week!

2: Breakfast: Low Carb Living beyond the Quiche

Even if you recognize the genius of the quiche, let's be realistic: if you eat the same breakfast, day after day, you will start having nightmares about it.

That easy slice of quiche that you are used to heating up in the morning might start showing up when you're asleep, trying to cram YOU into the microwave. Soon that donut shop that you drive by each morning on the way to work will start to beckon you even more seductively than it already does.

So what to do? The good news is that there are many low carb breakfast recipes that do not involve a mixture of eggs and cheese. This chapter gives you some other ideas for that first meal of the day. Prep time varies widely, which gives you a lot of choices no matter how little time you have to get breakfast ready on a particular day.

Pancakes (Yes, pancakes!) – Gluten-Free Coconut and Cinnamon Pancakes

This looks like a traditional pancake, but it's actually a hybrid of a pancake and an omelet. If you're starting to go through breakfast carb withdrawals, though, this is something to help you fight the cravings. You'll find these are a little heavier and drier than the pancakes you grew up eating, but they're definitely a real shot in the arm to keep you on the ketogenic path.

Ingredients:
2 large eggs
3 tablespoons full fat coconut milk
½ mashed ripe banana (about 2 tablespoons)
½ teaspoon apple cider vinegar
½ teaspoon vanilla extract
1½ tablespoons of organic coconut flour
½ teaspoon cinnamon
¼ teaspoon baking soda
1 small pinch of salt
Ghee or coconut oil (for frying)

Directions:

1. Whisk the mashed banana, coconut milk, eggs, vanilla extract and apple cider vinegar together, blending well.

2. Mix the other ingredients (but not the ghee) in a separate bowl.

3. Now whisk the wet and dry ingredients together right before you start cooking.

4. Put a tablespoon of ghee or coconut oil into a small skillet, and add a tablespoon of the batter.

5. Flip the pancake over as soon as you see bubbles forming on the top.

6. Allow to cook for about 30 more seconds, and then remove it.

7. Serve and enjoy!

Cauliflower Breakfast Hash

No, you don't have to use potatoes to make hash anymore. Instead, you can use cauliflower to get a similar flavor, but you end up with none of the gluten and only a handful of carbs instead. You can plop a runny yolk from a sunny side up egg right on top for a delicious breakfast.

Ingredients:
2 tablespoons olive oil
¾ lb. cauliflower, chopped into small segments

1 medium onion, diced
¼ teaspoon salt
¼ teaspoon smoked paprika
1/8 teaspoon black pepper
3 tablespoons water
2 teaspoons fresh parsley leaves, minced (for garnish)
2 teaspoons lemon juice
1 large clove garlic, minced

Directions

1. Place a large skillet over medium high heat, and heat the oil. Add an even layer of onion and cauliflower, and allow to cook without stirring until you see a bit of color on the bottom, so approximately 2 or 3 minutes.

2. Stir the mixture, and then add the water and spices. Cover and cook until the cauliflower becomes tender for the fork without being mushy and has turned gold, so approximately 3 to 5 minutes.

3. Bring the heat to low, and add in the garlic. Cook for 2 minutes, stirring the whole time.

4. Stir in the lemon juice and allow to cook until it evaporates, approximately half a minute.

5. Sprinkle the parsley on top (if desired), and put a fried egg on top as well, if you want one.

Low Carb Breakfast Burrito

One of the most delicious breakfast creations out there is the breakfast burrito. However, that flour tortilla is a real no-no for people on the ketogenic diet, and even the corn tortilla represents unnecessary carbohydrates. With just a little creativity, though, you can make your own breakfast burrito that does not rely on carbs to hold it together.

Ingredients:
2 eggs
Sliced ham (note: make sure it is thick and large enough to wrap around your food without breaking)
1/r cup chopped vegetables (such as tomato, black olives, bell peppers, spinach, and so on)
Salsa (optional)
Guacamole (optional)
Directions

1. Put a medium skillet over medium high heat, and add some oil before sautéing the vegetables.

2. Whisk the eggs in a small bowl and then pour over the mixed vegetables.

3. Scramble the mix in your skillet with a spatula until cooked, and remove the eggs from the pan.

4. Roll the slices of ham around the eggs, and put back into the skillet. Grill for 15 to 30 seconds on each side, slightly browning the ham.

5. Serve with guacamole and/or salsa as desired.

What do all of these breakfast choices have in common? They're relatively easy to make, and they are all friendly to the ketogenic diet. Remember – the key is keeping your carbs low and your protein high. This sort of breakfast will keep you full longer throughout your morning, so you'll be able to walk by that box of bagels in the break room without sending your body back to burning carbohydrates.

These breakfasts are also based on breakfast favorites. Pancakes are a breakfast favorite for many people growing up, and hash browns and burritos are often high on people's lists as well. While the ketogenic diet is not about tricking yourself, it is beneficial to find ways to let yourself enjoy what you eat. That way you won't see the diet as a burden – instead, you'll see it as an opportunity to change your lifestyle in a positive way.

3: The Mid-Morning Snack

Here's the deal: There are times when you'll head off track on a ketogenic diet when you're nowhere near mealtime. When temptation strikes and you end up going carb-crazy to the point where you tell yourself, perhaps for the millionth time, "I'll start that ketogenic thing TOMORROW."

The reason for this is that snacks are all around us, but they're not usually on a ketogenic plan. If you head into the break room at work, you're likely to find a machine filled with chips, candy bars and even gum.

You might see a package of peanuts or almonds, too, but it's not likely that they're going to tempt you as much as, say, that Kit-Kat bar or that bag of Doritos. So before you know it, you end up putting in your money and ripping open that package.

Why aren't there many ketogenic-friendly snacks in those machines? First of all, the processed sugars that form the backbone of many of those snacks are crucial when it comes to keeping them from going bad.

Many ketogenic snacks need to be refrigerated until you're ready to eat them, and the only time you'll find a chilled snack machine is when it is so cold that it stores ice cream and other frozen treats – again, things that aren't really on the ketogenic list of things to eat.

The recipes in this chapter are designed to help you get through those times in the day when your breakfast has already been digested but it's not time to think about lunch, and late at night when your stomach is rumbling but you don't really feel like getting out a skillet or turning on the grill to make something ketogenic-friendly.

Gluten-Free Strawberry Nutty Bars

It's all right if you want something sweet now and then. After all, if you didn't, you'd be missing out on a high percentage of your taste buds. But instead of grabbing that strawberry kolache from your co-worker's desk, reach for one of these.

Ingredients:
2 ¼ cups almond flour
¾ teaspoon baking soda
¾ teaspoon cinnamon
¾ teaspoon salt
½ cup equivalent granular sweetener
2 chia eggs
½ cup nut butter, melted slightly

¾ teaspoon vanilla
3 tablespoons dairy free milk

Topping:
1 teaspoon cinnamon
2 tablespoons equivalent sweetener
2 tablespoons coconut oil
½ cup unsweetened coconut flakes, chopped
1 cup pecans, chopped
¾ cup strawberry jam

Jam:
2 cups strawberries, halved
Equivalent sweetener to taste
2 tablespoons water
1 ½ tablespoons chia seeds

Instructions:
To make the jam, blend the water, sweetener and strawberries until the mixture is smooth. Pour this into a bowl and then add the chia seeds. Stir to mix and chill for at least 30 minutes, until it is set.

1. Preheat your oven to 350 F.

2. Combine all the dry bar ingredients in a medium to large bowl.

3. Combine the wet ingredients in a separate bowl, and then add the mixture to the dry ingredient bowl.

4. Mix thoroughly, and then press the blend into a square pan that you have already lined with some parchment paper.

5. Spread the jam evenly over all of the bars.

6. Make the topping by combining all of the ingredients into a bowl, mixing well, and then sprinkling on top of the jam.

7. Bake for about 20 minutes, covering with foil if you notice the topping darkening too much.

8. Remove from the oven to cool, and then put in the refrigerator for an hour or so.

Berries and Yogurt

This might be the easiest snack in the entire cookbook. You don't need a bunch of ingredients, and you don't have to follow a bunch of steps. Instead, pick your favorite berries out from the store: strawberries, blackberries, blueberries, raspberries, or whatever berries you want.

You can even get a variety if that's what you like. Layer them in a bowl with plain, unsweetened yogurt, and you have an easy snack that puts some pep in your morning.

Apples and Peanut Butter (or Almond Butter, or…you get it)

Again, here's another really easy snack recipe. Get one of your favorite apples (red, green, yellow, it's up to you). Slice it vertically, stopping when you hit the core but then moving to the other side. Pick up two of the slices, and spread peanut butter in between them to make a miniature sandwich.

To make it even more snazzy, put some chopped pecans or walnuts on a plate. Once you've added the peanut butter, put the top piece of apple on and press down so that just a little peanut butter oozes out through the sides. Then roll the sandwich through the chopped pecans so that they stick to the peanut butter. If you're not into peanut butter, almond butter works just as well.

Avocado Green Tea Power Shake

Want to give your morning a real jolt? Try this shake that is packed full of protein and antioxidants to help you get through to lunchtime feeling full and focused.

Ingredients:
1 tablespoon hot water
1 teaspoon matcha green tea powder
½ cup Greek yogurt (low-calorie)
¼ cup vanilla whey protein powder
½ medium avocado
2 teaspoons equivalent sweetener
1 ¼ cups unsweetened almond milk

Directions:

1. Whisk the hot water and matcha powder together in a small bowl, and put to one side.

2. Cut the avocado into chunks and put into the blender. Add the sweetener, protein powder and yogurt.

3. Add the tea mixture and almond milk, and then blend until the mixture is smooth.

4. You'll have enough for two glasses. Enjoy!

Try one of these snacks the next time you're facing one of those mid-morning lulls and just need to eat something to feel recharged. That way you won't feel that guilt that comes from licking the last of that Danish off your fingers. Instead, you'll still be on the way to teaching your body to burn fat and to leave carbs behind.

4: Lunch on the Go

This chapter is all about making lunches that you can eat on the go. This is a meal that often sends ketogenic dieters off their plan, because it's so much easier to go through the drive through lane or go out to a restaurant that serves carb-heavy meals. Try these ideas when you need a snappy lunch.

Get your meat ready ahead of time.

Remember that it's all about protein and fats with the ketogenic diet. Boil some eggs so that you have them in the fridge when you want a snack, or grab a few to make part of your lunch. Cook some bacon to the point where it's crispy, and keep it in the fridge so you can grab it for a snack.

Precook servings of salmon or another fatty fish (between 5 and 7 ounces), chicken thighs or turkey (3 to 4 ounces), or a few servings of slow cooked meat (up to 2 pounds) using a slow cooker and adding herbs like onion, rosemary and garlic. These can be the bases for very quick lunches.

Now for some recipes…
Prosciutto and Egg Roll-Ups

Ingredients:
1-2 eggs
Prosciutto

Directions:

1. Whisk the egg(s) in a bowl.

2. Melt a bit of butter or oil in a small skillet on high heat. Make sure you have enough egg to cover the entire bottom of the skillet, and add it before you bring the heat to low.

3. Wait for the egg to set, and then flip it over to cook it for about 30 more seconds.

4. Put the egg on your plate. Put a slice or two of prosciutto (or whatever meat you want). Then roll it up. Cut the rolls in half and put a toothpick in to hold them together. Now they're portable!

Asparagus and Chicken Lemon Stir Fry

Ingredients:
1 ½ pounds skinless chicken breast, cubed into 1-inch pieces

½ cup reduced sodium chicken broth
2 tablespoons water
2 tablespoons reduced sodium soy sauce
2 teaspoons cornstarch
1 bunch asparagus, ends removed, sliced into 2-inch segments
6 cloves garlic, chopped
1 tablespoon grape-seed oil, divided
1 tablespoon fresh ginger
3 tablespoons fresh lemon juice
Kosher salt and fresh black pepper, to taste

Directions:

1. Use the salt to lightly season the chicken. Combine the chicken broth and the soy sauce in a small bowl. Mix the water and cornstarch in a second small bowl, mixing well to blend.

2. Heat a large nonstick wok on medium high heat. When the wok is hot, add a teaspoon of the oil as well as the asparagus, cooking until tender and crisp, for about three or four minutes. Add the ginger and garlic and cook until the asparagus is golden, so about a minute. Put to one side.

3. Turn the heat up to high, and add a teaspoon of oil along with half the chicken. Cook until the chicken is thoroughly cooked and browned, approximately 4 minutes per side. Remove and put to one side, repeating with the rest of the chicken and oil. Put to one side.

4. Add in the soy sauce mixture, and bring it to a boil for cooking about 1 ½ minutes. Add the cornstarch mixture and the lemon juice, being sure to stir well. As it simmers, put the asparagus and chicken back in the wok and mix thoroughly. Take off the heat and serve.

Light Eggplant Parmesan with Salsa

Ingredients:
2 large aubergines
100 grams Parmesan cheese, finely grated
2 eggs
75 grams of almonds, chopped finely
2 garlic cloves, chopped finely
Coconut oil
Salt and pepper, to taste

For the salsa:
2 large tomatoes

1 avocado
1 red onion
2 tablespoons lemon juice2 tablespoons olive oil
2 tablespoons capers (if desired)
Fresh grated pepper, to taste

Directions:

1. Slice the aubergines lengthwise before rubbing coarse salt onto them. Allow them to sit for up to an hour. Rinse beneath cold water, and pat them dry using a kitchen cloth.

2. Whisk the eggs with pepper and salt within a deep dish. Mix the garlic, almond and Parmesan in another deep dish.

3. Heat the coconut oil in a skillet. Dip the slices of aubergine into the egg mixture and allow to trip before coating with the Parmesan mixture. Put them into the hot skillet one at a time. Fry on medium heat on both sides until they are golden and tender.

4. To make the salsa, dice the tomatoes, onion and avocado into small cubes. Chop fresh

basil (if desired) and mix it all together. Add the lemon juice, olive oil and pepper to taste.

5. Plate by setting a slice of aubergine in the bottom, covered with a layer of salsa, followed by another slice of aubergine, and finishing with the rest of the salsa. Top with an extra sprinkle of Parmesan.

Turkey and Hummus Lettuce Wraps

Ingredients:
4 leaves iceberg lettuce
½ cucumber, sliced
250 grams hummus
4 slices roast turkey
Paprika, to taste

Directions:

1. Unroll a lettuce leaf, and place a slice of turkey topped with cucumber, hummus and paprika. Then add a second piece of lettuce as though you were making a sandwich. Then roll up, and secure with a toothpick.

2. Repeat Step 1 until you have used all of the ingredients.

Not quite tasty enough? With this sort of recipe you can add other ingredients as well. Try some bell peppers, avocado or tomatoes. If you don't want turkey, try some prawns, grilled lamb, grilled chicken or grilled salmon. White cheeses also make a fine accompaniment as well.

These recipes are designed to help you make lunch that are easy to make and carry with you on a busy day. When your co-workers want to run through the drive-through or go out for a big lunch, you will have the weapons to resist their temptation sitting in that work refrigerator.

5: A More Relaxed Lunch

Obviously, not every lunch will be rushed. On the weekends, or on a lazy day off, cooking can be a relaxing pastime. Try these lighter recipes on those days when you have all the time you need to make the lunch that you want.

Bacon-Wrapped Mini Meat Loaves

Ingredients:
1 pound Ground beef
1 pound Bacon
2 garlic cloves, minced
¼ cup coconut milk
Parsley, chopped
1/3 cup fresh chives, minced
Black pepper, to taste

Directions:

1. Preheat the oven to 400 F.

2. Cut half of the slices of bacon into small chunks, and mix them with the ground beef, chives, garlic and coconut milk in a large bowl. Mix until the ingredients stick together.

3. Season this mixture with the black pepper to taste.

4. Take the remaining slices of bacon and put them around the sides of the holes in a muffin tin.

5. Add the beef mixture to the holes that have bacon in them.

6. Put the tin into the oven and let it cook for 30 minutes.

7. Remove from the oven and allow it to cool. Sprinkle with fresh parsley before serving.

Awesome Chili Cheese Dogs

That's right – just because you're giving up carbs doesn't mean you have to give up a favorite like this. You don't get to use buns anymore, but with these yams, you'll get the same great flavor.

Ingredients:
3 sweet potatoes, sliced lengthwise in half
6 hot dogs
1 pound ground beef

1 15 oz. can of fire roasted tomatoes, liquid drained, finely chopped
½ red onion, diced
2 cloves garlic, minced
1 tablespoon chili powder
½ teaspoon cocoa powder
3 oz. raw sharp cheddar cheese, grated
Salt and pepper to taste

Directions:

1. Preheat the oven to 450 F.

2. Spray the sweet potato slices with olive oil baking spray, and then place them on a baking sheet. Roast them for about half an hour.

3. Add a couple tablespoons of olive oil to a sauté pan. When it is hot, add garlic and onions, sautéing for about 10 minutes, until soft. Add the cocoa powder, chili powder, tomatoes, and chopped chipotle peppers, as well as the salt and pepper.

4. Crumble the beef into the sauté pan, breaking up large pieces. Allow the beef to cook through, simmering until the rest is done.

5. After the sweet potatoes are ready, take them off the baking sheet, and put the hot dogs on that same sheet. Put them in the oven and cook for about seven minutes, until they blister.

6. Grate the cheese, and scoop the meat out of the yams. You can use the sweet potato meat for other tasty meals. Now put the skin on a plate, with a hot dog on top of it. Spoon on some chili and add some grated cheese to the top.

Enchilada Chicken Mango Salad

Ingredients:
1 small head of hearts of romaine, shredded
1 mango, peeled and diced
2 cups cold leftover enchilada chicken
½ avocado, diced
Salt and pepper to taste

Directions:

1. Chop up the romaine lettuce.

2. Put the chicken on top.

3. Add the avocado and mango.

4. Serve

Chef Salad Ham Cups

Ingredients:
2 slices ham, thinly sliced
Lettuce, shredded
Tomato, shredded
Hard boiled egg, chopped
Cheddar cheese, shredded

Directions:

1. Preheat the oven to 350 F.

2. Put a muffin pan or custard cups on a cookie sheet.

3. Put two slices of ham over an inverted muffin pan or custard cup, in the shape of an X.

4. Put another custard cup over the first to keep the ham from burning.

5. Cut any extra ham from the bottom, leaving an inch or so.

6. Bake for 20 minutes.

7. Take out of the oven carefully, and allow it to cool.

8. Take the top bowl off to cool, and then remove the bottom bowl.

9. Add shredded cheese and lettuce, as well as the chopped egg and tomato, to the cups. Serve cold.

NOTE: You'll need two slices of ham for each cup.

Shrimp and Avocado Salad

Ingredients:
Dressing/Marinade:
3 tablespoons fresh lime juice
½ cup fresh cilantro, chopped
2 tablespoons extra virgin olive oil
Salt and black pepper, to taste

Salad:

Cilantro dressing
2 ripe avocados
1 pound cooked shrimp, tail removed and deveined
4 cups baby greens or lettuce

Directions:

1. Pour the marinade over the shrimp; if you are using thawed shrimp, be sure to pour off any excess water. Stir to coat the shrimp evenly, and cover and refrigerate for at least an hour.

2. Wash and dry the lettuce, and divide among the plates.

3. Cut the avocado into small wedges and sprinkle over the lettuce.

4. Top with any leftover dressing and the marinated shrimp.

Asian-Inspired Chicken Wings

Ingredients:
3 pounds chicken wings, separated
2 tablespoons extra virgin coconut oil
1 tablespoon fresh ginger, chopped
4 cloves fresh garlic, chopped

1 teaspoon fennel seed
1 teaspoon anise seed
½ cup coconut aminos
2 tablespoons coconut vinegar
2 tablespoons honey
2 tablespoons sesame oil
1 tablespoon fish sauce

Directions:

1. Put the chicken wings in a large bowl, patting dry if necessary.

2. Heat the coconut oil over medium high heat in a small pan. Add fennel and anise seed, garlic and ginger and cook, stirring frequently to keep from burning, about two minutes.

3. Add honey, coconut aminos, fish sauce and vinegar. Heat to a boil and allow simmering for one minute.

4. Take off the heat, and add sesame oil.

5. Pour on top the chicken wings, stirring to coat. Once the wings are cool enough to touch, cover them and put them in the

refrigerator to marinate as long as 24 hours. Stir them once or twice while marinating to ensure even coverage.

6. Drain any excess marinade. Barbecue them, turning them once; this should take about 20 minutes, depending on the grill. You can also bake them for 45 minutes or an hour at 375 F.

6: Rock the Afternoon Snack

A couple of hours after lunch, it's not uncommon to feel a bit of a lull. This is a time when it's really easy to reach for a donut or head to the break room and raid the fridge. Instead, have some snacks on hand to keep your cravings at bay.

Before we get to the recipes, here is a list of some snack foods to keep on hand. You don't have to have a refrigerator to keep these fresh.

Almonds
Pecans
Peanuts
Kale chips
Beef jerky
Turkey jerky

Now, for some snack recipes

Almond Thins

Ingredients:
3 oz. almond flour
2 teaspoons granular Splenda
1 egg white
3/8 teaspoon salt
1/8 teaspoon onion powder

1/8 teaspoon garlic powder

Directions:

1. Preheat oven to 325 F.

2. Mix the ingredients thoroughly in a small bowl, until the dough sticks together.

3. Grease a sheet of aluminum foil, and arrange the dough on it, crumbling the mixture and spreading it in a rectangular shape. Cover the dough with wax paper that you have sprayed with a non-stick coating.

4. Roll the dough to a thickness no more than 1/8 inch, making it even.

5. Remove the wax paper, and use a ravioli or pizza cutter to cut the dough into squares an inch per side.

6. Set the foil on the oven rack, and bake until the squares are golden brown, about 10 or 15 minutes. Check after 10 minutes and take out any crackers with browned edges.

Throwback Protein Bars

Ingredients:
1 pound grass fed beef heart or flank steak
2 cups kale, chopped
4 cups frozen spinach, chopped
2 cups wild blueberries
½ cup dried apricots
¼ cup extra virgin coconut oil
½ cup tallow

Directions:

1. Slice the beef into ¼-inch thick pieces and arrange on a tray inside a food dehydrator.

2. Dehydrate the meat for at least five hours, until it is firm and mostly devoid of moisture.

3. Place the kale and spinach onto a fruit roll sheet inside your food dehydrator, and do the same with the blueberries.

4. Dehydrate for at least three hours, until the blueberries are chewy and small and the greens are absolutely crisp. The meat should be crisp as well.

5. Place the greens and meat into a food processor and grind as finely as you can.

6. Process the apricots finely in your food processor.

7. Melt the tallow and coconut oil.

8. Mix the apricot, blueberries, meat and greens in a bowl. Add the tallow and coconut oil, stirring until it all holds together. Add a tablespoon of coconut oil if it is not sticky enough.

9. Push the mixture into a square pan. Chill until it firms, and then cut into bars.

Homemade Beef Jerky

Ingredients:
1 pound ground beef
1 teaspoon salt
1 teaspoon pepper (more if you want a spicier product)

Directions:

1. Mix the ground beef with your seasonings until it is all well blended.

2. Pipe jerky onto food dehydrator trays with an extruder.

3. Dehydrate the beef for at least six hours. Try to find the point where the beef will almost break in half.

4. Set the trays into the oven to allow the meat to dry. If it is still fairly moist, preheat the oven to its lowest setting.

5. Remove and store.

Sweet and Salty Fudge Bombs

1 cup whole walnuts or pecans
1 1/3 cups dates, pitted (about 16)
1 teaspoon vanilla extract
4 tablespoons cocoa powder
Sea salt to garnish
Unsweetened, shredded coconut to garnish

Directions:

1. Put the cocoa powder, vanilla, dates and nuts into a food processor. Process at high speed until you achieve a paste with a glossy, smooth texture.

2. Put water on your hands, and shake off any extra. Then form one-inch balls out of the dough. Place on a baking sheet.

3. Put a couple tablespoons of sea salt on a plate, dipping the top of the bombs. Just get a few grains to adhere to the top.

4. For coconut, put shredded coconut on the plate and roll each ball in it, pressing the coconut into the ball with your hands.

5. Chill the bombs in the refrigerator for 30 minutes to an hour to add firmness.

Homemade Kale Chips

Ingredients:
8 cups kale (loosely packed), ripped into 1-inch pieces, stems removed
2 tablespoons extra virgin coconut oil melted and warm - Salt to taste

Directions:

1. Preheat oven to 325 F.

2. Wash the kale, patting to dry. Set in a large bowl.

3. Pour the warm oil on top of the kale. Place a lid on the bowl, and shake to coat. You can also stir them to coat.

4. Spread the pieces of kale on a large baking sheet, and then sprinkle with just a bit of salt.

5. Bake for 20 minutes, until the chips are crispy.

Cheese Roll-ups

Ingredients:
2 ounces mozzarella cheese, shredded
Pizza or marinara sauce
Garlic powder

Directions:

1. Spread the cheese across the bottom of a nonstick skillet, making sure to cover the entire pan. Put the range on medium high heat.

2. Sprinkle the cheese with garlic powder to taste.

3. Start prying the cheese up with a spatula once the bottom becomes a golden brown.

4. Roll the edge of the cheese toward the middle with the spatula, and then put the roll onto a plate.

5. Serve with a bowl of marinara or pizza sauce as a dipping option.

These snacks are all guaranteed to be easy to keep on hand. If you have these in your drawer at work, you're much more likely to be able to avoid those afternoon cravings that can send your diet over the edge of a cliff. Use these ketogenic-friendly recipes to satisfy the need for a little bit of food while keeping your carb counts extremely low.

7: Quick dinner recipes for on the Go

Families seem to get busier and busier with each passing year. Kids have more activities in which they take part, and with both parents often working, the name of the game is often ease and convenience when dinnertime rolls around.

This means too many meals purchased from a drive-through window – and packed with sodium and the wrong kinds of fat, as well as loads of carbs.
If you need to grab your dinner and go, you can still eat the ketogenic way, but you have to do some planning ahead.

The recipes in this section are all possible to cook ahead of time and freeze, or prepare in a snap so that you don't have to spend much time slaving over a hot stove.

Pizza Toppings Casserole

Ingredients:
8 ounces fresh mushrooms, sliced
4 eggs
1 pound bulk Italian sausage
¼ cup pizza sauce (recipe below)
½ cup heavy cream

1/2 teaspoon basil
¼ teaspoon garlic powder
3 ½ ounces pepperoni, chopped
½ cup bell pepper, chopped
½ cup red onion, slivered
8 ounces whole milk mozzarella cheese, cubed

Directions:

1. Brown the mushrooms and sausage, draining the grease afterward.

2. Whisk the cream, seasonings, pizza sauce and eggs in a medium bowl.

3. Grease a baking dish and add the peppers, mushrooms, meats and cheese cubes. Then, pour the egg mixture in, mixing thoroughly. Put the red onion on top.

4. Sprinkle some more seasonings on top, as well as some crushed red pepper if you are so inclined.

5. Preheat the oven to 350 F.

6. Bake the casserole for 45 to 55 minutes until you see a nice browning, and you can slide a knife into the center and bring it out cleanly.

7. Remove from the oven and allow standing for about five minutes.

Pizza Sauce Recipe
1 8 ounce can tomato sauce
2 tablespoons tomato paste
½ cup water
2 teaspoons granular Splenda
¼ teaspoon garlic powder
½ teaspoon dried basil

Directions:

Bring all of these ingredients to boil in a small. Cover the pot partially and simmer for about an hour over low heat.

Southern Barbecue Meatballs

Ingredients:
Meatballs
1 pound ground pork
1 teaspoon paprika
1 teaspoon granulated Splenda

¼ teaspoon black pepper
½ teaspoon salt
¼ teaspoon cayenne pepper
¼ teaspoon celery salt
½ teaspoon ground cumin
¼ cup almond flour
1 egg
1 tablespoon water

Sauce:
2 teaspoons hot sauce
¼ cup yellow mustard
1 tablespoon dried onion flakes
2 tablespoons apple cider vinegar
2 tablespoons low sugar ketchup
3 tablespoons granulated Splenda
Salt and pepper to taste

Directions:

Sauce:

1. Put all of the ingredients together into a small saucepan, stirring to achieve a smooth consistency.

2. Turn the heat on low, and allow simmering for 8 to 10 minutes.

Meatballs:

1. Place all of the meatball ingredients into a medium sized bowl and mix completely. Form the blend into 16 meatballs. In a large sauté pan, fry the meatballs at medium heat until they look golden on each side, giving about 3 minutes per side.

2. Toss the meatballs in the sauce, and then spread on a baking sheet lined in parchment.

3. Turn on the broiler, and place the meatballs inside for 2 to 3 minutes.

Cheesy Tuna Casserole

Ingredients:
2 6 oz. cans of tuna, drained
1 pound frozen French cut green beans
3 oz. fresh mushrooms, chopped
1 stalk celery, chopped finely
2 tablespoons onion, chopped finely
½ cup chicken broth
2 tablespoons butter
¾ cup heavy cream
Salt and pepper to taste
4 to 8 oz. cheddar cheese, shredded

Directions:

1. Follow the directions on the package of green beans to cook them in a medium pot. While that is cooking, sauté the onion, celery and mushrooms in the butter until they are quite soft and are just beginning to brown.

2. Add the broth to the sauté pan, and bring the whole thing to a boil. When the liquid has reduced by half, stir the cream in, and bring back to a boil.

3. Reduce the heat and cook until the mixture has thickened and reduced, stirring often.

4. Season to taste, and then stir the mushroom soup mixture and tuna in to the green beans. Spice to taste.

5. Mix the cheese in, and then put the whole dish into a casserole. Bake at 350 F until the casserole is hot and bubbling.

Low Carb Fish Sticks

Ingredients:
1 ½ pounds haddock (or any fish that is meaty, white and firm)
6 oz. plantain chips
Coconut oil

Directions:

1. Crunch the plantain chips up in a food processor until they look like fine crumbs of bread.

2. Put the crumbs into a Ziploc bag with a touch of salt. Then, shake the bag gently.

3. Slice the fish into sticks or planks. Place a few into the bag and shake, coating them completely.

4. Add coconut oil to your sauté pan and turn on medium heat. Place the strips in the pan, and brown them on each side, about a minute or less on each side.

Roasted Baby Carrots (side dish)

Ingredients:
1 pound baby carrots
1 tablespoon oil
¼ to ½ teaspoon salt, to taste

Directions:

1. Line a baking pan with nonstick foil.

2. Place carrots in the pan, drizzling oil across the top. Sprinkle salt to taste.

3. Preheat the oven to 475 F.

4. Roast the carrots for 10 to 12 minutes. Stir, and bake for four more minutes, and stir once again.

5. Bake for four more minutes, stopping when the carrots are browned and tender.

All of the recipes in this chapter are designed to help you stay on the ketogenic plan, even when your family has a busy night. The casseroles will keep all week in the freezer, so if you prepare them on Sunday and thaw them out during the week, you'll have a home-cooked meal without all of the cooking and cleanup.

8: Dinner Recipes for Relaxed Evenings

Hopefully not EVERY night in your home is a series of road rallies from one activity to the next. There's nothing better than sitting down to a warm, tasty meal. Try one of these recipes the next time you have a while to prepare dinner and savor it with your family or friends.

Bacon Wrapped Scallops

Ingredients:
12 scallops
12 slices of microwaveable bacon
12 toothpicks
1 tablespoon oil
Salt and pepper to taste

Directions:

1. Put a skillet on high heat, and add a tablespoon of oil.

2. Wrap a piece of bacon around each scallop, and use a toothpick to hold it in place.

3. Season with salt and pepper to taste.

4. Cook for two or three minutes on each side.

Butter Pork Kabobs

Ingredients:
Marinade:
3 tablespoons sunflower butter
1 tablespoon soy sauce
2 teaspoons hot sauce
1 tablespoon garlic, minced
½ teaspoon crushed red pepper
1 tablespoon water

Pork Kabobs:
1 pound pork kabob squares
1 medium green bell pepper

Directions:

1. Put all of the marinade ingredients into a food processor, and mix until you have a smooth texture.

2. Slice the pork into bite sized squares, and put them into a bowl.

3. Mix the marinade and pork together and soak for 1 to 24 hours.

4. Chop the bell pepper up into small slices.

5. Thread the pork and bell pepper onto metal skewers.

6. Broil the kebabs on high for 5 minutes on each side. Internal temperature should be at least 145 F.

Oodles with Lamb Meatballs

Ingredients:
2 pounds zucchini
1 pound pasta sauce
1 pound ground lamb
1 egg yolk
2 shallots
1 teaspoon cumin
1 teaspoon cinnamon
Cayenne pepper, salt and black pepper to taste

Directions:

1. Preheat the oven to 450 F.

2. Run the zucchini through a mandolin set to julienne, stopping when you get to the seeded part.

3. Mix the other ingredients together (except for the pasta sauce) to make 16 meatballs.

4. Place the meatballs on a baking sheet, and put in the oven for 12 minutes.

Put the zoodles, pasta sauce and meatballs into a saucepan, and cook on medium high for 3 or 4 minutes.

St. Louis Ribs

Ingredients:
2 racks of St. Louis ribs
2 tablespoons granulated Splenda
2 tablespoons paprika
1 tablespoon salt
1 tablespoon garlic powder
½ tablespoon pepper
½ tablespoon ginger, ground
½ tablespoon onion powder
¼ tablespoon cayenne pepper
2 oz. Dijon mustard

Directions:

1. Preheat the oven to 225 F.

2. Take the membrane from the back of the rib rack with a sharp knife.

3. Mix the spices all together.

4. Cover the ribs with mustard, making sure to spread evenly.

5. Rub the mixture of spices into the mustard and meat.

6. Line a baking sheet with foil, and place the ribs on it.

7. Bake without covering for an hour.

8. Use aluminum foil to make a tent over the meat, and then cook for 3 to 3 ½ more hours, turning after two hours. Internal temperature should be 180 F.

9. Take the foil tent off and broil on high for 4 to 6 minutes to make a crust. Then cover and put to one side to rest for 8 to 10 minutes.

Bacon Explosion

Ingredients:
29 slices bacon, thick cut
14 oz. steak
10 oz. pork sausage
4 oz. cheddar cheese, shredded

Directions:

1. Lay out a weaved pattern of bacon, 5 x 6. Preheat oven to 400 F, and bake the weave for 15 minutes or so, until it is almost crisp.

2. Grind bacon, sausage and steak together to make a meat mixture.

3. Lay the meat mixture out in a rectangle that is the same size as the weave of bacon.

4. Season the mixture, and then put the bacon weave on the meat.

5. Put the cheese in the center of the bacon.

6. Make a tight roll out of the meat, and then put in the refrigerator.

7. Now make a 7 x 7 bacon weave.

8. Roll the bacon weave over the meat diagonally.

9. Bake at 400 F for 50 minutes to an hour. Internal temperature should be 165 F. Allow to set for 10 minutes before slicing.

Loaded Baked Chicken

Ingredients:
4 strips of bacon
4 chicken breasts, boneless and skinless
1 oz. soy sauce
4 oz. ranch dressing
4 oz. cheddar cheese
3 green onions

Directions:

1. Place some cooking oil into a skillet, and turn the heat on high.

2. Fry the chicken breasts in the skillet, flipping after five or six minutes. When the internal temperature hits 165 F, they are ready to come out.

3. Prepare bacon bits while the chicken is in the skillet by cooking the bacon and crumbling it.

4. Chop 3 green onion stalks.

5. Put the chicken into a baking dish, and put soy sauce on top of it. Then, add ranch, bacon, green onions and the cheddar cheese.

6. Place on the broiler, at high heat, for three or four minutes, until the cheese melts.

Curry Chicken with Riced Cauliflower

Ingredients:
1 packet curry paste
2 pounds of chicken

1 cup water
3 tablespoons ghee or butter
½ cup heavy cream
1 cauliflower head

Directions:

1. Melt the butter or ghee in a large pan or pot. Add the curry paste and stir to mix.

2. Add water and simmer for about five minutes.

3. Add chicken, cover, and simmer for 20 minutes. During this time, chop the head of cauliflower into its florets, and put it into the food processor on Pulse to create riced cauliflower.

4. After the chicken is finished, take the cover off, add cream and cook for five minutes. Serve over the riced cauliflower.

All of the meals in this chapter are warm and enticing. You won't walk away from the table missing all of the carbs that you could have had. Instead, you will enjoy the symphony of flavors in each. Best of all, you'll still be teaching your body to turn to fat for its energy instead of sugar.

9: Time for Dessert!

The health benefits of the ketogenic diet are numerous. However, when it comes to dessert, this eating plan is second to none. Take a look at some of these treats – even though they are low on carbs, you will love the way they taste!

Coconut Macaroons

Ingredients:
1 teaspoon vanilla
4 egg whites
½ teaspoon granulated Splenda
4 ½ teaspoons water
2 cups unsweetened coconut

Directions:

1. Mix the egg whites, vanilla and water.

2. Add the coconut and Splenda and mix together.

3. Spread the mixture on a greased pie pan.

4. Preheat the oven to 375 F. Turn the heat down to 325 F when you put the pan in the oven.

5. Bake for 12 to 14 minutes.

Strawberry Cheesecake

Ingredients:
Crust:
¾ cup almond flour
¾ cup pecans
2 tablespoons granulated Splenda
4 tablespoons butter

Filling:
4 eggs
1 ½ pounds cream cheese
½ tablespoon liquid vanilla
½ tablespoon lemon juice
1 cup Splenda
¼ cup sour cream
9 strawberries

Directions:

1. Preheat the oven to 400 F. Crush the pecans. Melt the butter in a small saucepan, and add the crust's Splenda, almond flour and pecans.

2. Mix the crust for several minutes in the saucepan until the texture is consistent.

3. Grease a springform pan and use the crust to line the bottom.

4. Cook for 7 minutes until the crust starts to turn brown.

5. Combine all of the filling ingredients except the strawberries in a mixing bowl, and mix thoroughly.

6. Slice strawberries and use them to line the side of the crust.

7. Add the filling on top of the strawberries and crust. Put the cheesecake in the oven at 400F but turn the temperature down to 250F right when you place it in.

8. Cook for 1 to 1 ½ hours, or until the cheesecake sets.

9. Allow the cheesecake to cool, and then keep it in the refrigerator until you are ready to serve it.

Mint Chocolate Chip Ice Cream

Ingredients:
½ cup light cream
1 cup heavy cream
½ teaspoon liquid Stevia extract
½ teaspoon vanilla
1 square dark chocolate

Several drops of peppermint extract and green food coloring

Directions:

1. Follow the instructions of your ice cream maker regarding how long you should put the bowl in the freezer ahead of time; this is usually somewhere between 4 and 12 hours.

2. Put all of the ingredients except the chocolate square into a metal bowl, and whisk thoroughly.

3. Place the bowl back in the freezer for 5 minutes.

4. Set up the ice cream maker per the manufacturer's instructions.

5. Shave the chocolate square, and add the shavings a couple of minutes before the ice cream set.

6. Store in an airtight container, and put in the freezer.

Strawberry Chocolate Mousse

Ingredients:
1/3 cup heavy whipping cream
4 drops EZ-SWEET
1 strawberry
½ scoop chocolate whey powder
90% chocolate flakes

Directions:

1. Measure the cream into a container

2. Add the EZ-SWEET, strawberry and whey powder

3. Add the chocolate flakes, and mix for a minute or two, until it's stiff

4. Serve, refrigerating any leftovers

Lemon Squares

Ingredients:

Crust:
1 cup almond flour, fine ground
¼ teaspoon sea salt
1 tablespoon coconut oil, melted
2 tablespoons raw unsalted butter, melted
2 tablespoons powdered xylitol
1 tablespoon pure vanilla extract

Topping:
¼ cup powdered xylitol
¼ cup almond flour, fine ground
4 large eggs
2 teaspoons spoonable Stevia
½ cup fresh squeezed lemon juice

Directions:

1. Preheat the oven to 350F. Line a baking dish with parchment paper.

2. For the crust, combine the xylitol, almond flour and sea salt in a large bowl. Stir together the butter, vanilla and coconut oil in a smaller bowl. Stir the wet mixture into the dry, combining thoroughly. Push the dough into the baking dish evenly. Bake for 12 to 15 minutes, stopping when the crust has a light gold color.

3. For the topping, whisk the xylitol, almond flour, eggs, stevia and lemon juice until they are smooth. Take the crust out of the oven when it is finished, and pour the topping over it evenly while the crust is still hot.

4. Put the pan back into the oven, and bake for 15 to 20 minutes at 350 F. Take it out when the topping turns golden on the edges. Allow to cool in its baking dish for a half hour, and then put it in the refrigerator for two hours to

set. Sprinkle with more xylitol as desired. Slice into bars.

Berry Cream Cheese Tart

Ingredients:
Crust:
1 tablespoon granulated brown Splenda
¼ cup almond meal
¼ teaspoon salt
2/3 cup walnut pieces
1 tablespoon coconut oil, melted
1 tablespoon water
1 egg white

Filling:
8 oz. cream cheese
½ cup granulated Stevia
3 eggs
½ teaspoon vanilla
2/3 cup half and half
3 tablespoons lemon juice
4 oz. each of blueberries, raspberries and blackberries
Zest from 1 lemon

Directions:
1. Preheat your oven to 350 F. Pulse the brown sugar, salt, walnuts, coconut oil and almond

meal until you have a finely processed mixture. Press the mixture evenly into a tart dish.

2. Mix the water and egg white together, brushing the crust lightly with it. Bake for 15 to 18 minutes or until the crust is a golden brown. Take out of the oven, cool for a few minutes, and then put in the freezer for 15 minutes.

3. Turn the oven down to 325 F. Beat the cream cheese until it is smooth, and add the sweetener before mixing until you have consistent texture.

4. Mix in the eggs, one at a time. Then slowly add the vanilla, half and half, lemon zest and lemon juice, mixing until they have disappeared into the mixture.

5. Pour the mixture into the crust, and bake for half an hour, or when you can shake the dish without the mixture moving much at all.

6. Cool in the refrigerator, and use the berries to top when you are ready to serve.

These desserts all come in handy when you need to satiate your sweet tooth. Put these to work when you have a family or occasion where you need a decadent flavor without a decadent number of carbs.

10: Head to the Soup Counter

Soup is a great meal for people who are on a diet. With the right composition, a soup can be a filling meal. However, the high liquid content means that you can feel satisfied without having to eat as bulky a dinner.

Cheesy Tortilla Soup

Ingredients:
1 envelope chicken fajita seasoning mix
2 tablespoons canola oil
1 pound boneless skinless chicken breasts, diced
½ cup chopped onion
¼ cup butter, cubed
2 cans (14 ½ oz. each) chicken broth
1/3 cup all-purpose flour
1/3 cup canned diced tomatoes with chilies
1 cup cubed processed cheese
1 ½ cups half and half cream
1 ½ cups shredded Monterey Jack cheese, divided
½ cup shredded cheddar cheese

Guacamole and tortilla chips

Directions:

1. Follow the directions on the package for the fajita mix, and then add the chicken before marinating as instructed. Cook the chicken in a large skillet with the oil until the chicken is not pink any more, and set aside.

2. Sauté the onion in butter inside a large saucepan until the onion is tender. Stir flour in until it is all blended. Stir broth in gradually, and bring to a boil. Cook while stirring for 2 minutes or until you see bubbles and thickening. Add the tomatoes, 1 cup of the Monterey Jack and the processed cheese. Stir and cook until all of the cheese melts.

3. Stir the cream and reserved chicken in, heating through without boiling. Sprinkle the cheddar and the rest of the Monterey Jack cheese. Put chips and guacamole on top to complete the presentation.

Crab Soup with Sherry

Ingredients:
1 pound frozen or fresh crabmeat
6 tablespoons chicken broth or sherry

¼ cup butter, cubed
1 small onion, grated
¼ cup all-purpose flour
2 cups 2% milk
½ teaspoon salt
2 chicken bouillon cubes
3 cups half and half cream
2 tablespoons fresh parsley, minced

Directions:

1. Mix the sherry and crabmeat in a small bowl, and then set aside.

2. Sauté the onion in butter in a large saucepan until the onion is tender.

3. Stir in salt and flour until they blend, and then add bouillon and milk. Bring to a boil before stirring and cooking for 2 minutes or until it thickens. Stir in the crab and cream mixture before heating through. Sprinkle parsley on the servings.

Cabbage Soup

Ingredients:
1 teaspoon pepper

1 teaspoon salt
1 tablespoon garlic
1 packet onion soup mix
4 cups chopped carrots
2 cups chopped celery
5 cloves garlic
6 cups chicken broth
4 slices of mushroom
1 head cabbage
2 cups chopped bell pepper
1 pound of onion

Directions:

1. Add the olive oil to a large stock pot that you have on medium heat.

2. Add in the garlic, onions and peppers, and heat until you can see through the onions.

3. Add the mushrooms and celery.

4. Add the soup mix, carrots, spices and chicken stock.

5. Bring the mixture to a boil, and then turn down low to simmer.

6. Add the cabbage now, pushing it into the liquid and adding filtered water to cover the cabbage.

7. Cook for an hour, and allow cooling before you serve it.

Traditional Egg Drop Soup

Ingredients:
1 tablespoon soy sauce
1 tablespoon corn starch
¼ teaspoon white pepper
4 cups chicken stock
3 large eggs, beaten slightly
½ teaspoon ginger, grated
¾ cup pieces of baby bella mushrooms
3 stalks green onion, chopped

Directions:

1. Reserve ½ cup of the stock, and mix in with the cornstarch until it dissolves.

2. Put the ginger, chicken stock, green onions, mushrooms, white pepper and soy sauce into a pot, and heat to a boil.

3. Add the stock mixture and cornstarch before stirring. Turn the heat down to a simmer.

4. Add in those beaten eggs while you slowly stir the soup. The egg tends to spread out in ribbons.

Low Carb Broccoli Cheese Soup

Ingredients:
2 cups cheddar cheese, shredded
1 small package cream cheese
2 cans chicken broth
1 cup fluid heavy cream
1 package chopped broccoli

Directions:

1. Put a pot over medium high heat and heat the chicken broth inside it.

2. In another bowl, mix the cream cheese, cheddar cheese, heavy cream and 2 tablespoons of butter (if desired). Microwave for 30 second intervals to see if it softens enough. Stir each time you check on the butter.

3. After the broth gets hot, stir the frozen broccoli in before heating the soup again.

4. After the soup is heated, add the cream cheese mixture with the chicken broth and broccoli. Keep stirring in order to melt these cheeses.

5. Turn the burner off when the soup is hot again, and place half the broccoli along with ¼ cup of broth into a blender for pureeing. This gives your soup a thicker texture and makes it taste creamier.

6. Pour the puree back into the pot before stirring it well. Serve hot, garnishing with cheese if you desire.

Tomato Soup

Ingredients
10 plum tomatoes
1 teaspoon black pepper
1 tablespoon olive oil
1 tablespoon tarragon leaves
1 clove garlic
1 cube bouillon (low sodium)
2 tbsp. shallots, chopped

4 cups water

Directions:

1. Heat the oil over medium high heat in a nonstick saucepan.

2. Add the shallots and garlic before cooking 5 minutes, until they are softer and start to turn brown.

3. Cut the tomatoes into large pieces, and add into the saucepan.

4. Sprinkle the tarragon over the tomatoes.

5. Sauté tomatoes for five minutes.

6. Add 4 cups of water along with the bouillon cube.

7. Simmer for 20 minutes.

8. Run the soup through a blender before serving.

Conclusion

Over the years, many different weight loss strategies have come and gone. In the final analysis, losing weight comes down to just one simple formula: calories in and calories out. If you take in more calories than you burn, you will gain weight; if you burn more than you take in, the pounds will come off.

The ketogenic diet represents a chance to make a change in the entire way your body approaches food. By getting your body off of sugar as its fuel source, the ketogenic diet revolutionizes our relationship with carbohydrates.

The agrarian lifestyle gave us an unhealthy association with grains over time. Add that to the breakfast cereal phenomenon that began in Battle Creek, Michigan, around the turn of the century, and you have an obsession with carbohydrates that has come to plague waistlines all over the West.

Modern diets simply contain way too many carbohydrates. If you look up and down the menu of many mainstream restaurants, you will see entrees and lists of sides that are heavy on processed sugars. It is true that the restaurateurs are just giving us what we want, but what we want has more than doubled in size over the past decades.

The ketogenic diet has given many people a new lease on life. Their clothes fit better, they have more energy – and they don't have to give up their favorite flavors (who could imagine a world without bacon, for example?)

By eating this way, you prepare your body to deal with fats much more efficiently. This means that your body will store less fat, and your metabolism will go through a much flatter curve during the day, keeping you from having those big lulls in the morning and afternoon.

Enjoy the recipes in this book!

Printed in Great Britain
by Amazon.co.uk, Ltd.,
Marston Gate.